PERSONAL INFORMATION

Name:	
Address:	**City:**
	Home Phone #:
State/Zip:	**Mobile No #:**

GENDER | M | F

BLOOD GROUP

HEIGHT

WEIGHT

BMI

EMERGENCY CONTACTS

Name:	
Address:	**City:**
	Home Phone #:
State/Zip:	**Mobile No #:**
Relationship:	

D1530139

Name:	
Address:	**City:**
	Home Phone #:
State/Zip:	**Mobile No #:**
Relationship:	

FAMILY MEDICAL HISTORY

MEDICAL CONDITION	FAMILY MEMBER	NOTES
High Blood Pressure:		
Diabetes		
High Cholesterol		
Heart Disease		
Stroke/TIA		
Allergies		
Auto Immune Diseases		
Cancer		
Arthritis		
Birth Defects		
Infertility		
Mental Illness		
Kidney Disease		
Liver Disease		
Lung Disease		
Blood Disorder		
Gastrointestinal Disorder		
Nerve Disorders		
Migraines		
Endometriosis		

MEDICAL CONTACTS

Doctor:

Phone:

Dentist:

Phone:

Eye Doctor:

Phone:

Pharmacy:

Phone:

MEDICAL HEALTH HISTORY

Allergies

1:	
2:	
3:	
4:	

Major Illnesses

1:	
2:	
3:	
4:	
5:	

Surgeries

Date:	
Type:	

Date:	
Type:	

Date:	
Type:	

Date:	
Type:	

MEDICINE

Medication	Dosage	Treatment	Start	End	Note

MEDICINE

Medication	Dosage	Treatment	Start	End	Note

☑ DATE [ ]

DAILY CARE	✓	GROOMING	BATHING	EATING	GETTING DRESSED
	Self				
	With Help				
	Caregiver				

MEALS	BREAKFAST	LUNCH	DINNER
	TIME		

SNACKS	AM SNACKS	PM SNACKS

OTHERS	DRINKS	OTHERS

DAILY CARE	TIME	MEDICATION TAKEN

BUSY TIME	PHONE CALLS & VISITS	ACTIVITIES

	WATER INTAKE	
	SLEEP	

DOCTORS VISIT	SPECIALIST	COMMENTS

TOILET	URINE					
	BOWEL					
	NOTES					

PHYSICAL PAIN	PAIN LOCATION	MARK 1-5

NOTES

VITALS		MORNING	MID-DAY	NIGHT
	Blood Sugar			
	Blood Pressure			
	Oxygen Level			
	Heart Rate			

OVERALL	HOW WAS THE DAY?
	AWESOME GOOD OK DOWN PAINFUL
	REMARKS

☑ DATE _____

DAILY CARE	✓	GROOMING	BATHING	EATING	GETTING DRESSED
	Self				
	With Help				
	Caregiver				

MEALS	BREAKFAST	LUNCH	DINNER
	TIME		

SNACKS	AM SNACKS	PM SNACKS

OTHERS	DRINKS	OTHERS

DAILY CARE	TIME	MEDICATION TAKEN

BUSY TIME	PHONE CALLS & VISITS	ACTIVITIES

DOCTORS VISIT	SPECIALIST	COMMENTS

PHYSICAL PAIN	PAIN LOCATION	MARK 1-5

VITALS	MORNING	MID-DAY	NIGHT
Blood Sugar			
Blood Pressure			
Oxygen Level			
Heart Rate			

OVERALL

HOW WAS THE DAY?

AWESOME	GOOD	OK	DOWN	PAINFUL

REMARKS

WATER INTAKE

SLEEP

TOILET						
URINE						
BOWEL						

NOTES

NOTES

☑ DATE

DAILY CARE	✓	GROOMING	BATHING	EATING	GETTING DRESSED
	Self				
	With Help				
	Caregiver				

MEALS	BREAKFAST	LUNCH	DINNER
TIME			

SNACKS	AM SNACKS	PM SNACKS

OTHERS	DRINKS	OTHERS

DAILY CARE	TIME	MEDICATION TAKEN

BUSY TIME

PHONE CALLS & VISITS	ACTIVITIES

DOCTORS VISIT

SPECIALIST	COMMENTS

PHYSICAL PAIN

PAIN LOCATION	MARK 1-5

VITALS

	MORNING	MID-DAY	NIGHT
Blood Sugar			
Blood Pressure			
Oxygen Level			
Heart Rate			

OVERALL

HOW WAS THE DAY?

:D AWESOME	:) GOOD	:| OK	:(DOWN	:((PAINFUL

REMARKS

WATER INTAKE

SLEEP

TOILET

URINE					
BOWEL					

NOTES

NOTES

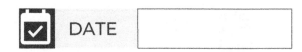

DATE

DAILY CARE	✓	GROOMING	BATHING	EATING	GETTING DRESSED
	Self				
	With Help				
	Caregiver				

MEALS	BREAKFAST	LUNCH	DINNER
	TIME		

SNACKS	AM SNACKS	PM SNACKS

OTHERS	DRINKS	OTHERS

DAILY CARE	TIME	MEDICATION TAKEN

BUSY TIME	PHONE CALLS & VISITS	ACTIVITIES

DOCTORS VISIT	SPECIALIST	COMMENTS

PHYSICAL PAIN	PAIN LOCATION	MARK 1-5

VITALS	MORNING	MID-DAY	NIGHT
Blood Sugar			
Blood Pressure			
Oxygen Level			
Heart Rate			

OVERALL — HOW WAS THE DAY?

AWESOME	GOOD	OK	DOWN	PAINFUL

REMARKS

WATER INTAKE

SLEEP

TOILET						
URINE						
BOWEL						

NOTES

NOTES

 DATE

DAILY CARE

✔	GROOMING	BATHING	EATING	GETTING DRESSED
Self				
With Help				
Caregiver				

MEALS

	BREAKFAST	LUNCH	DINNER
TIME			

SNACKS

AM SNACKS	PM SNACKS

OTHERS

DRINKS	OTHERS

DAILY CARE

TIME	MEDICATION TAKEN

BUSY TIME	PHONE CALLS & VISITS	ACTIVITIES

	WATER INTAKE	

	SLEEP	

DOCTORS VISIT	SPECIALIST	COMMENTS

TOILET	URINE					
	BOWEL					
	NOTES					

PHYSICAL PAIN	PAIN LOCATION	MARK 1-5

NOTES

VITALS		MORNING	MID-DAY	NIGHT
	Blood Sugar			
	Blood Pressure			
	Oxygen Level			
	Heart Rate			

OVERALL	HOW WAS THE DAY?
	AWESOME GOOD OK DOWN PAINFUL
	REMARKS

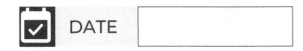 DATE

DAILY CARE	✓	GROOMING	BATHING	EATING	GETTING DRESSED
	Self				
	With Help				
	Caregiver				

MEALS	BREAKFAST	LUNCH	DINNER
	TIME		

SNACKS	AM SNACKS	PM SNACKS

OTHERS	DRINKS	OTHERS

DAILY CARE	TIME	MEDICATION TAKEN

BUSY TIME	PHONE CALLS & VISITS	ACTIVITIES

	WATER INTAKE	
	SLEEP	

DOCTORS VISIT	SPECIALIST	COMMENTS

TOILET	URINE					
	BOWEL					
	NOTES					

PHYSICAL PAIN	PAIN LOCATION	MARK 1-5

NOTES

VITALS		MORNING	MID-DAY	NIGHT
	Blood Sugar			
	Blood Pressure			
	Oxygen Level			
	Heart Rate			

OVERALL	HOW WAS THE DAY?
	AWESOME GOOD OK DOWN PAINFUL
	REMARKS

DATE [ ]

DAILY CARE	✓	GROOMING	BATHING	EATING	GETTING DRESSED
	Self				
	With Help				
	Caregiver				

MEALS	BREAKFAST	LUNCH	DINNER
	TIME		

SNACKS	AM SNACKS	PM SNACKS

OTHERS	DRINKS	OTHERS

DAILY CARE	TIME	MEDICATION TAKEN

BUSY TIME

PHONE CALLS & VISITS	ACTIVITIES

DOCTORS VISIT

SPECIALIST	COMMENTS

PHYSICAL PAIN

PAIN LOCATION	MARK 1-5

VITALS

	MORNING	MID-DAY	NIGHT
Blood Sugar			
Blood Pressure			
Oxygen Level			
Heart Rate			

OVERALL

HOW WAS THE DAY?

😃 AWESOME	🙂 GOOD	😐 OK	🙁 DOWN	😣 PAINFUL

REMARKS

WATER INTAKE

SLEEP

TOILET

URINE					
BOWEL					

NOTES

NOTES

DATE

DAILY CARE	✓	GROOMING	BATHING	EATING	GETTING DRESSED
	Self				
	With Help				
	Caregiver				

MEALS		BREAKFAST	LUNCH	DINNER
	TIME			

SNACKS	AM SNACKS	PM SNACKS

OTHERS	DRINKS	OTHERS

DAILY CARE	TIME	MEDICATION TAKEN

BUSY TIME	PHONE CALLS & VISITS	ACTIVITIES

	WATER INTAKE	

	SLEEP	

DOCTORS VISIT	SPECIALIST	COMMENTS

TOILET	URINE					
	BOWEL					

NOTES

PHYSICAL PAIN	PAIN LOCATION	MARK 1-5

NOTES

VITALS		MORNING	MID-DAY	NIGHT
	Blood Sugar			
	Blood Pressure			
	Oxygen Level			
	Heart Rate			

OVERALL	HOW WAS THE DAY?

AWESOME	GOOD	OK	DOWN	PAINFUL

REMARKS

DATE

DAILY CARE	✓	GROOMING	BATHING	EATING	GETTING DRESSED
	Self				
	With Help				
	Caregiver				

MEALS		BREAKFAST	LUNCH	DINNER
	TIME			

SNACKS	AM SNACKS	PM SNACKS

OTHERS	DRINKS	OTHERS

DAILY CARE	TIME	MEDICATION TAKEN

BUSY TIME	PHONE CALLS & VISITS	ACTIVITIES

DOCTORS VISIT	SPECIALIST	COMMENTS

PHYSICAL PAIN	PAIN LOCATION	MARK 1-5

VITALS		MORNING	MID-DAY	NIGHT
	Blood Sugar			
	Blood Pressure			
	Oxygen Level			
	Heart Rate			

OVERALL

HOW WAS THE DAY?

☺ AWESOME	☺ GOOD	☺ OK	☹ DOWN	☹ PAINFUL

REMARKS

WATER INTAKE

SLEEP

TOILET							
URINE							
BOWEL							
NOTES							

NOTES

☑ DATE [ ]

DAILY CARE

✓	GROOMING	BATHING	EATING	GETTING DRESSED
Self				
With Help				
Caregiver				

MEALS

	BREAKFAST	LUNCH	DINNER
TIME			

SNACKS

AM SNACKS	PM SNACKS

OTHERS

DRINKS	OTHERS

DAILY CARE

TIME	MEDICATION TAKEN

BUSY TIME	PHONE CALLS & VISITS	ACTIVITIES

WATER INTAKE	
SLEEP	

TOILET							
	URINE						
	BOWEL						
NOTES							

DOCTORS VISIT	SPECIALIST	COMMENTS

NOTES

PHYSICAL PAIN	PAIN LOCATION	MARK 1-5

VITALS		MORNING	MID-DAY	NIGHT
	Blood Sugar			
	Blood Pressure			
	Oxygen Level			
	Heart Rate			

OVERALL	HOW WAS THE DAY?
	AWESOME GOOD OK DOWN PAINFUL
	REMARKS

☑ DATE [   ]

DAILY CARE	✓	GROOMING	BATHING	EATING	GETTING DRESSED
	Self				
	With Help				
	Caregiver				

MEALS		BREAKFAST	LUNCH	DINNER
	TIME			

SNACKS	AM SNACKS	PM SNACKS

OTHERS	DRINKS	OTHERS

DAILY CARE	TIME	MEDICATION TAKEN

BUSY TIME	PHONE CALLS & VISITS	ACTIVITIES

DOCTORS VISIT	SPECIALIST	COMMENTS

PHYSICAL PAIN	PAIN LOCATION	MARK 1-5

VITALS		MORNING	MID-DAY	NIGHT
	Blood Sugar			
	Blood Pressure			
	Oxygen Level			
	Heart Rate			

OVERALL	HOW WAS THE DAY?
	☺ AWESOME ☺ GOOD 😐 OK ☹ DOWN ☹ PAINFUL
	REMARKS

WATER INTAKE

SLEEP

TOILET	URINE						
	BOWEL						
	NOTES						

NOTES

 DATE [ ]

DAILY CARE

✓	GROOMING	BATHING	EATING	GETTING DRESSED
Self				
With Help				
Caregiver				

MEALS

TIME	BREAKFAST	LUNCH	DINNER

SNACKS

AM SNACKS	PM SNACKS

OTHERS

DRINKS	OTHERS

DAILY CARE

TIME	MEDICATION TAKEN

BUSY TIME	PHONE CALLS & VISITS	ACTIVITIES

	WATER INTAKE	
	SLEEP	

DOCTORS VISIT	SPECIALIST	COMMENTS

TOILET	URINE					
	BOWEL					
	NOTES					

PHYSICAL PAIN	PAIN LOCATION	MARK 1-5

NOTES

VITALS		MORNING	MID-DAY	NIGHT
	Blood Sugar			
	Blood Pressure			
	Oxygen Level			
	Heart Rate			

OVERALL	HOW WAS THE DAY?
	AWESOME GOOD OK DOWN PAINFUL
	REMARKS

DATE ☑

✓	GROOMING	BATHING	EATING	GETTING DRESSED
Self				
With Help				
Caregiver				

DAILY CARE

MEALS

BREAKFAST	LUNCH	DINNER
TIME		

SNACKS

AM SNACKS	PM SNACKS

OTHERS

DRINKS	OTHERS

DAILY CARE

TIME	MEDICATION TAKEN

BUSY TIME	PHONE CALLS & VISITS	ACTIVITIES

WATER INTAKE	
SLEEP	

TOILET	URINE					
	BOWEL					
	NOTES					

DOCTORS VISIT	SPECIALIST	COMMENTS

NOTES

PHYSICAL PAIN	PAIN LOCATION	MARK 1-5

VITALS		MORNING	MID-DAY	NIGHT
	Blood Sugar			
	Blood Pressure			
	Oxygen Level			
	Heart Rate			

OVERALL	HOW WAS THE DAY?
	AWESOME GOOD OK DOWN PAINFUL
	REMARKS

☑ **DATE** [ ]

DAILY CARE	✓	GROOMING	BATHING	EATING	GETTING DRESSED
	Self				
	With Help				
	Caregiver				

MEALS		BREAKFAST	LUNCH	DINNER
	TIME			

SNACKS	AM SNACKS	PM SNACKS

OTHERS	DRINKS	OTHERS

DAILY CARE	TIME	MEDICATION TAKEN

BUSY TIME	PHONE CALLS & VISITS	ACTIVITIES

	WATER INTAKE	

	SLEEP	

DOCTORS VISIT	SPECIALIST	COMMENTS

TOILET	URINE					
	BOWEL					
	NOTES					

PHYSICAL PAIN	PAIN LOCATION	MARK 1-5

NOTES

VITALS		MORNING	MID-DAY	NIGHT
	Blood Sugar			
	Blood Pressure			
	Oxygen Level			
	Heart Rate			

OVERALL	HOW WAS THE DAY?
	AWESOME GOOD OK DOWN PAINFUL
	REMARKS

DATE [ ]

DAILY CARE	✓	GROOMING	BATHING	EATING	GETTING DRESSED
	Self				
	With Help				
	Caregiver				

MEALS	BREAKFAST	LUNCH	DINNER
	TIME		

SNACKS	AM SNACKS	PM SNACKS

OTHERS	DRINKS	OTHERS

DAILY CARE	TIME	MEDICATION TAKEN

BUSY TIME

PHONE CALLS & VISITS	ACTIVITIES

DOCTORS VISIT

SPECIALIST	COMMENTS

PHYSICAL PAIN

PAIN LOCATION	MARK 1-5

VITALS

	MORNING	MID-DAY	NIGHT
Blood Sugar			
Blood Pressure			
Oxygen Level			
Heart Rate			

OVERALL

HOW WAS THE DAY?

☺ AWESOME	☺ GOOD	😐 OK	☹ DOWN	🙁 PAINFUL

REMARKS	

WATER INTAKE

SLEEP

TOILET

URINE					
BOWEL					

NOTES

NOTES

☑ DATE

DAILY CARE

✓	GROOMING	BATHING	EATING	GETTING DRESSED
Self				
With Help				
Caregiver				

MEALS

	BREAKFAST	LUNCH	DINNER
TIME			

SNACKS

AM SNACKS	PM SNACKS

OTHERS

DRINKS	OTHERS

DAILY CARE

TIME	MEDICATION TAKEN

BUSY TIME	PHONE CALLS & VISITS	ACTIVITIES

WATER INTAKE	
SLEEP	

TOILET							
URINE							
BOWEL							
NOTES							

DOCTORS VISIT	SPECIALIST	COMMENTS

PHYSICAL PAIN	PAIN LOCATION	MARK 1-5

VITALS	MORNING	MID-DAY	NIGHT
Blood Sugar			
Blood Pressure			
Oxygen Level			
Heart Rate			

NOTES

OVERALL	HOW WAS THE DAY?

AWESOME	GOOD	OK	DOWN	PAINFUL

REMARKS

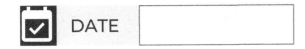 DATE

DAILY CARE	✔	GROOMING	BATHING	EATING	GETTING DRESSED
	Self				
	With Help				
	Caregiver				

MEALS	BREAKFAST	LUNCH	DINNER
	TIME		

SNACKS	AM SNACKS	PM SNACKS

OTHERS	DRINKS	OTHERS

DAILY CARE	TIME	MEDICATION TAKEN

BUSY TIME	PHONE CALLS & VISITS	ACTIVITIES

	WATER INTAKE	
	SLEEP	

DOCTORS VISIT	SPECIALIST	COMMENTS

TOILET	URINE					
	BOWEL					
	NOTES					

PHYSICAL PAIN	PAIN LOCATION	MARK 1-5

NOTES

VITALS		MORNING	MID-DAY	NIGHT
	Blood Sugar			
	Blood Pressure			
	Oxygen Level			
	Heart Rate			

OVERALL	HOW WAS THE DAY?
	AWESOME GOOD OK DOWN PAINFUL
	REMARKS

☑ **DATE**

DAILY CARE	✔	GROOMING	BATHING	EATING	GETTING DRESSED
	Self				
	With Help				
	Caregiver				

MEALS	BREAKFAST	LUNCH	DINNER
	TIME		

SNACKS	AM SNACKS	PM SNACKS

OTHERS	DRINKS	OTHERS

DAILY CARE	TIME	MEDICATION TAKEN

BUSY TIME	PHONE CALLS & VISITS	ACTIVITIES

DOCTORS VISIT	SPECIALIST	COMMENTS

PHYSICAL PAIN	PAIN LOCATION	MARK 1-5

VITALS	MORNING	MID-DAY	NIGHT
Blood Sugar			
Blood Pressure			
Oxygen Level			
Heart Rate			

OVERALL

HOW WAS THE DAY?

AWESOME	GOOD	OK	DOWN	PAINFUL

REMARKS

WATER INTAKE

SLEEP

TOILET							
URINE							
BOWEL							
NOTES							

NOTES

☑ DATE [   ]

DAILY CARE	✓	GROOMING	BATHING	EATING	GETTING DRESSED
	Self				
	With Help				
	Caregiver				

MEALS	BREAKFAST	LUNCH	DINNER
	TIME		

SNACKS	AM SNACKS	PM SNACKS

OTHERS	DRINKS	OTHERS

DAILY CARE	TIME	MEDICATION TAKEN

BUSY TIME

PHONE CALLS & VISITS	ACTIVITIES

DOCTORS VISIT

SPECIALIST	COMMENTS

PHYSICAL PAIN

PAIN LOCATION	MARK 1-5

VITALS

	MORNING	MID-DAY	NIGHT
Blood Sugar			
Blood Pressure			
Oxygen Level			
Heart Rate			

OVERALL

HOW WAS THE DAY?

AWESOME	GOOD	OK	DOWN	PAINFUL

REMARKS

WATER INTAKE

SLEEP

TOILET

URINE					
BOWEL					

NOTES

NOTES

DATE [   ]

DAILY CARE

✔	GROOMING	BATHING	EATING	GETTING DRESSED
Self				
With Help				
Caregiver				

MEALS

	BREAKFAST	LUNCH	DINNER
TIME			

SNACKS

AM SNACKS	PM SNACKS

OTHERS

DRINKS	OTHERS

DAILY CARE

TIME	MEDICATION TAKEN

BUSY TIME	PHONE CALLS & VISITS	ACTIVITIES

DOCTORS VISIT	SPECIALIST	COMMENTS

PHYSICAL PAIN	PAIN LOCATION	MARK 1-5

VITALS	MORNING	MID-DAY	NIGHT
Blood Sugar			
Blood Pressure			
Oxygen Level			
Heart Rate			

OVERALL

HOW WAS THE DAY?

😃 AWESOME 🙂 GOOD 😐 OK 🙁 DOWN 😖 PAINFUL

REMARKS

WATER INTAKE

SLEEP

TOILET							
URINE							
BOWEL							

NOTES

NOTES

☑ DATE [ ]

DAILY CARE	✓	GROOMING	BATHING	EATING	GETTING DRESSED
	Self				
	With Help				
	Caregiver				

MEALS	BREAKFAST	LUNCH	DINNER
	TIME		

SNACKS	AM SNACKS	PM SNACKS

OTHERS	DRINKS	OTHERS

DAILY CARE	TIME	MEDICATION TAKEN

BUSY TIME	PHONE CALLS & VISITS	ACTIVITIES

	WATER INTAKE	

	SLEEP	

DOCTORS VISIT	SPECIALIST	COMMENTS

TOILET	URINE					
	BOWEL					
	NOTES					

PHYSICAL PAIN	PAIN LOCATION	MARK 1-5

NOTES

VITALS		MORNING	MID-DAY	NIGHT
	Blood Sugar			
	Blood Pressure			
	Oxygen Level			
	Heart Rate			

OVERALL	HOW WAS THE DAY?
	AWESOME GOOD OK DOWN PAINFUL
	REMARKS

DATE ☑ [   ]

DAILY CARE	✓	GROOMING	BATHING	EATING	GETTING DRESSED
	Self				
	With Help				
	Caregiver				

MEALS		BREAKFAST	LUNCH	DINNER
	TIME			

SNACKS	AM SNACKS	PM SNACKS

OTHERS	DRINKS	OTHERS

DAILY CARE	TIME	MEDICATION TAKEN

BUSY TIME

PHONE CALLS & VISITS	ACTIVITIES

DOCTORS VISIT

SPECIALIST	COMMENTS

PHYSICAL PAIN

PAIN LOCATION	MARK 1-5

VITALS

	MORNING	MID-DAY	NIGHT
Blood Sugar			
Blood Pressure			
Oxygen Level			
Heart Rate			

OVERALL

HOW WAS THE DAY?

:D AWESOME	:) GOOD	:| OK	:(DOWN	:'(PAINFUL

REMARKS	

WATER INTAKE

SLEEP

TOILET

URINE					
BOWEL					

NOTES

NOTES

☑ DATE [ ]

DAILY CARE

✔	GROOMING	BATHING	EATING	GETTING DRESSED
Self				
With Help				
Caregiver				

MEALS

BREAKFAST		LUNCH	DINNER
TIME			

SNACKS

AM SNACKS	PM SNACKS

OTHERS

DRINKS	OTHERS

DAILY CARE

TIME	MEDICATION TAKEN

BUSY TIME

PHONE CALLS & VISITS	ACTIVITIES

DOCTORS VISIT

SPECIALIST	COMMENTS

PHYSICAL PAIN

PAIN LOCATION	MARK 1-5

VITALS

	MORNING	MID-DAY	NIGHT
Blood Sugar			
Blood Pressure			
Oxygen Level			
Heart Rate			

OVERALL

HOW WAS THE DAY?

:-D AWESOME	:-) GOOD	:-| OK	:-(DOWN	:-(PAINFUL

REMARKS

WATER INTAKE

SLEEP

TOILET

URINE					
BOWEL					

NOTES

NOTES

DATE [ ]

DAILY CARE	✔	GROOMING	BATHING	EATING	GETTING DRESSED
	Self				
	With Help				
	Caregiver				

MEALS	BREAKFAST	LUNCH	DINNER
	TIME		

SNACKS	AM SNACKS	PM SNACKS

OTHERS	DRINKS	OTHERS

DAILY CARE	TIME	MEDICATION TAKEN

BUSY TIME	PHONE CALLS & VISITS	ACTIVITIES

WATER INTAKE	

SLEEP	

DOCTORS VISIT	SPECIALIST	COMMENTS

TOILET	URINE					
	BOWEL					
NOTES						

PHYSICAL PAIN	PAIN LOCATION	MARK 1-5

NOTES

VITALS		MORNING	MID-DAY	NIGHT
	Blood Sugar			
	Blood Pressure			
	Oxygen Level			
	Heart Rate			

OVERALL	HOW WAS THE DAY?
	😃 AWESOME 🙂 GOOD 😐 OK 🙁 DOWN 😣 PAINFUL
	REMARKS

☑ **DATE** [   ]

DAILY CARE

✓	GROOMING	BATHING	EATING	GETTING DRESSED
Self				
With Help				
Caregiver				

MEALS

	BREAKFAST	LUNCH	DINNER
TIME			

SNACKS

AM SNACKS	PM SNACKS

OTHERS

DRINKS	OTHERS

DAILY CARE

TIME	MEDICATION TAKEN

BUSY TIME	PHONE CALLS & VISITS	ACTIVITIES

DOCTORS VISIT	SPECIALIST	COMMENTS

PHYSICAL PAIN	PAIN LOCATION	MARK 1-5

VITALS		MORNING	MID-DAY	NIGHT
	Blood Sugar			
	Blood Pressure			
	Oxygen Level			
	Heart Rate			

OVERALL

HOW WAS THE DAY?

☺ AWESOME   ☺ GOOD   😐 OK   ☹ DOWN   😖 PAINFUL

REMARKS

WATER INTAKE

SLEEP

TOILET							
	URINE						
	BOWEL						
	NOTES						

NOTES

DATE [ ]

DAILY CARE	✓	GROOMING	BATHING	EATING	GETTING DRESSED
	Self				
	With Help				
	Caregiver				

MEALS		BREAKFAST	LUNCH	DINNER
	TIME			

SNACKS	AM SNACKS	PM SNACKS

OTHERS	DRINKS	OTHERS

DAILY CARE	TIME	MEDICATION TAKEN

BUSY TIME	PHONE CALLS & VISITS	ACTIVITIES

WATER INTAKE	

SLEEP	

TOILET							
URINE							
BOWEL							
NOTES							

DOCTORS VISIT	SPECIALIST	COMMENTS

PHYSICAL PAIN	PAIN LOCATION	MARK 1-5

VITALS	MORNING	MID-DAY	NIGHT
Blood Sugar			
Blood Pressure			
Oxygen Level			
Heart Rate			

NOTES

OVERALL — HOW WAS THE DAY?

AWESOME   GOOD   OK   DOWN   PAINFUL

REMARKS

DATE [ ]

DAILY CARE	✓	GROOMING	BATHING	EATING	GETTING DRESSED
	Self				
	With Help				
	Caregiver				

MEALS		BREAKFAST	LUNCH	DINNER
	TIME			

SNACKS	AM SNACKS	PM SNACKS

OTHERS	DRINKS	OTHERS

DAILY CARE	TIME	MEDICATION TAKEN

BUSY TIME	PHONE CALLS & VISITS	ACTIVITIES

	WATER INTAKE	

	SLEEP	

DOCTORS VISIT	SPECIALIST	COMMENTS

TOILET	URINE						
	BOWEL						
	NOTES						

PHYSICAL PAIN	PAIN LOCATION	MARK 1-5

NOTES

VITALS		MORNING	MID-DAY	NIGHT
	Blood Sugar			
	Blood Pressure			
	Oxygen Level			
	Heart Rate			

OVERALL	HOW WAS THE DAY?
	AWESOME GOOD OK DOWN PAINFUL
	REMARKS

☑ DATE [   ]

DAILY CARE	✓	GROOMING	BATHING	EATING	GETTING DRESSED
	Self				
	With Help				
	Caregiver				

MEALS		BREAKFAST	LUNCH	DINNER
	TIME			

SNACKS	AM SNACKS	PM SNACKS

OTHERS	DRINKS	OTHERS

DAILY CARE	TIME	MEDICATION TAKEN

BUSY TIME	PHONE CALLS & VISITS	ACTIVITIES

DOCTORS VISIT	SPECIALIST	COMMENTS

PHYSICAL PAIN	PAIN LOCATION	MARK 1-5

VITALS		MORNING	MID-DAY	NIGHT
	Blood Sugar			
	Blood Pressure			
	Oxygen Level			
	Heart Rate			

OVERALL — HOW WAS THE DAY?

AWESOME · GOOD · OK · DOWN · PAINFUL

REMARKS

WATER INTAKE

SLEEP

TOILET							
	URINE						
	BOWEL						

NOTES

NOTES

☑ DATE [   ]

DAILY CARE	✓	GROOMING	BATHING	EATING	GETTING DRESSED
	Self				
	With Help				
	Caregiver				

MEALS	BREAKFAST	LUNCH	DINNER
	TIME		

SNACKS	AM SNACKS	PM SNACKS

OTHERS	DRINKS	OTHERS

DAILY CARE	TIME	MEDICATION TAKEN

BUSY TIME

PHONE CALLS & VISITS	ACTIVITIES

DOCTORS VISIT

SPECIALIST	COMMENTS

PHYSICAL PAIN

PAIN LOCATION	MARK 1-5

VITALS

	MORNING	MID-DAY	NIGHT
Blood Sugar			
Blood Pressure			
Oxygen Level			
Heart Rate			

OVERALL

HOW WAS THE DAY?

AWESOME	GOOD	OK	DOWN	PAINFUL

REMARKS

WATER INTAKE

SLEEP

TOILET

URINE					
BOWEL					

NOTES

NOTES

DATE ☑

DAILY CARE	✓	GROOMING	BATHING	EATING	GETTING DRESSED
	Self				
	With Help				
	Caregiver				

MEALS	BREAKFAST	LUNCH	DINNER
	TIME		

SNACKS	AM SNACKS	PM SNACKS

OTHERS	DRINKS	OTHERS

DAILY CARE	TIME	MEDICATION TAKEN

BUSY TIME

PHONE CALLS & VISITS	ACTIVITIES

DOCTORS VISIT

SPECIALIST	COMMENTS

PHYSICAL PAIN

PAIN LOCATION	MARK 1-5

VITALS

	MORNING	MID-DAY	NIGHT
Blood Sugar			
Blood Pressure			
Oxygen Level			
Heart Rate			

OVERALL

HOW WAS THE DAY?

AWESOME · GOOD · OK · DOWN · PAINFUL

REMARKS

WATER INTAKE

SLEEP

TOILET

URINE					
BOWEL					

NOTES

NOTES

☑ DATE [　　　　　　　]

DAILY CARE	✔	GROOMING	BATHING	EATING	GETTING DRESSED
	Self				
	With Help				
	Caregiver				

MEALS	BREAKFAST	LUNCH	DINNER
	TIME		

SNACKS	AM SNACKS	PM SNACKS

OTHERS	DRINKS	OTHERS

DAILY CARE	TIME	MEDICATION TAKEN

BUSY TIME

PHONE CALLS & VISITS	ACTIVITIES

DOCTORS VISIT

SPECIALIST	COMMENTS

PHYSICAL PAIN

PAIN LOCATION	MARK 1-5

VITALS

	MORNING	MID-DAY	NIGHT
Blood Sugar			
Blood Pressure			
Oxygen Level			
Heart Rate			

OVERALL

HOW WAS THE DAY?

:D AWESOME	:) GOOD	:| OK	:(DOWN	:'(PAINFUL

REMARKS	

WATER INTAKE

SLEEP

TOILET

URINE						
BOWEL						

NOTES

NOTES

DATE ☑ [_____]

DAILY CARE	✔	GROOMING	BATHING	EATING	GETTING DRESSED
	Self				
	With Help				
	Caregiver				

MEALS	BREAKFAST	LUNCH	DINNER
	TIME		

SNACKS	AM SNACKS	PM SNACKS

OTHERS	DRINKS	OTHERS

DAILY CARE	TIME	MEDICATION TAKEN

BUSY TIME	PHONE CALLS & VISITS	ACTIVITIES

WATER INTAKE

SLEEP

TOILET						
URINE						
BOWEL						
NOTES						

DOCTORS VISIT	SPECIALIST	COMMENTS

NOTES

PHYSICAL PAIN	PAIN LOCATION	MARK 1-5

VITALS	MORNING	MID-DAY	NIGHT
Blood Sugar			
Blood Pressure			
Oxygen Level			
Heart Rate			

OVERALL	HOW WAS THE DAY?
	😃 AWESOME 🙂 GOOD 😐 OK 🙁 DOWN 😣 PAINFUL
	REMARKS

☑ **DATE**

DAILY CARE	✔	GROOMING	BATHING	EATING	GETTING DRESSED
	Self				
	With Help				
	Caregiver				

MEALS		BREAKFAST	LUNCH	DINNER
	TIME			

SNACKS	AM SNACKS	PM SNACKS

OTHERS	DRINKS	OTHERS

DAILY CARE	TIME	MEDICATION TAKEN

BUSY TIME	PHONE CALLS & VISITS	ACTIVITIES

	WATER INTAKE	
	SLEEP	

DOCTORS VISIT	SPECIALIST	COMMENTS

TOILET	URINE					
	BOWEL					
	NOTES					

PHYSICAL PAIN	PAIN LOCATION	MARK 1-5

NOTES

VITALS		MORNING	MID-DAY	NIGHT
	Blood Sugar			
	Blood Pressure			
	Oxygen Level			
	Heart Rate			

OVERALL

HOW WAS THE DAY?

AWESOME	GOOD	OK	DOWN	PAINFUL

REMARKS	

☑ DATE

DAILY CARE	✔	GROOMING	BATHING	EATING	GETTING DRESSED
	Self				
	With Help				
	Caregiver				

MEALS		BREAKFAST	LUNCH	DINNER
	TIME			

SNACKS	AM SNACKS	PM SNACKS

OTHERS	DRINKS	OTHERS

DAILY CARE	TIME	MEDICATION TAKEN

BUSY TIME

PHONE CALLS & VISITS	ACTIVITIES

DOCTORS VISIT

SPECIALIST	COMMENTS

PHYSICAL PAIN

PAIN LOCATION	MARK 1-5

VITALS

	MORNING	MID-DAY	NIGHT
Blood Sugar			
Blood Pressure			
Oxygen Level			
Heart Rate			

OVERALL

HOW WAS THE DAY?

🙂 AWESOME	🙂 GOOD	😐 OK	🙁 DOWN	🙁 PAINFUL

REMARKS

WATER INTAKE

SLEEP

TOILET

URINE					
BOWEL					

NOTES

NOTES

DATE

DAILY CARE

✔	GROOMING	BATHING	EATING	GETTING DRESSED
Self				
With Help				
Caregiver				

MEALS

	BREAKFAST	LUNCH	DINNER
TIME			

SNACKS

AM SNACKS	PM SNACKS

OTHERS

DRINKS	OTHERS

DAILY CARE

TIME	MEDICATION TAKEN

BUSY TIME	PHONE CALLS & VISITS	ACTIVITIES

	WATER INTAKE	
	SLEEP	

DOCTORS VISIT	SPECIALIST	COMMENTS

TOILET	URINE					
	BOWEL					
	NOTES					

PHYSICAL PAIN	PAIN LOCATION	MARK 1-5

NOTES

VITALS		MORNING	MID-DAY	NIGHT
	Blood Sugar			
	Blood Pressure			
	Oxygen Level			
	Heart Rate			

OVERALL	HOW WAS THE DAY?
	AWESOME GOOD OK DOWN PAINFUL
	REMARKS

☑ **DATE** [ ]

DAILY CARE

✓	GROOMING	BATHING	EATING	GETTING DRESSED
Self				
With Help				
Caregiver				

MEALS

BREAKFAST	LUNCH	DINNER
TIME		

SNACKS

AM SNACKS	PM SNACKS

OTHERS

DRINKS	OTHERS

DAILY CARE

TIME	MEDICATION TAKEN

BUSY TIME	PHONE CALLS & VISITS	ACTIVITIES

WATER INTAKE	

SLEEP	

DOCTORS VISIT	SPECIALIST	COMMENTS

TOILET						
URINE						
BOWEL						
NOTES						

PHYSICAL PAIN	PAIN LOCATION	MARK 1-5

📝 **NOTES**

VITALS		MORNING	MID-DAY	NIGHT
	Blood Sugar			
	Blood Pressure			
	Oxygen Level			
	Heart Rate			

OVERALL — HOW WAS THE DAY?

AWESOME	GOOD	OK	DOWN	PAINFUL
😃	🙂	😐	🙁	😣

REMARKS

☑ DATE [   ]

DAILY CARE	✓	GROOMING	BATHING	EATING	GETTING DRESSED
	Self				
	With Help				
	Caregiver				

MEALS	BREAKFAST	LUNCH	DINNER
	TIME		

SNACKS	AM SNACKS	PM SNACKS

OTHERS	DRINKS	OTHERS

DAILY CARE	TIME	MEDICATION TAKEN

BUSY TIME	PHONE CALLS & VISITS	ACTIVITIES

	WATER INTAKE	
	SLEEP	

DOCTORS VISIT	SPECIALIST	COMMENTS

TOILET	URINE					
	BOWEL					
	NOTES					

PHYSICAL PAIN	PAIN LOCATION	MARK 1-5

NOTES

VITALS		MORNING	MID-DAY	NIGHT
	Blood Sugar			
	Blood Pressure			
	Oxygen Level			
	Heart Rate			

OVERALL	HOW WAS THE DAY?
	AWESOME GOOD OK DOWN PAINFUL
	REMARKS

☑ **DATE** [_____]

DAILY CARE	✓	GROOMING	BATHING	EATING	GETTING DRESSED
	Self				
	With Help				
	Caregiver				

MEALS		BREAKFAST	LUNCH	DINNER
	TIME			

SNACKS	AM SNACKS	PM SNACKS

OTHERS	DRINKS	OTHERS

DAILY CARE	TIME	MEDICATION TAKEN

BUSY TIME

PHONE CALLS & VISITS	ACTIVITIES

DOCTORS VISIT

SPECIALIST	COMMENTS

PHYSICAL PAIN

PAIN LOCATION	MARK 1-5

VITALS

	MORNING	MID-DAY	NIGHT
Blood Sugar			
Blood Pressure			
Oxygen Level			
Heart Rate			

OVERALL

HOW WAS THE DAY?

😃 AWESOME	🙂 GOOD	😐 OK	🙁 DOWN	😣 PAINFUL

REMARKS	

WATER INTAKE

SLEEP

TOILET

URINE					
BOWEL					

NOTES

NOTES

DATE ☑ [   ]

DAILY CARE

✔	GROOMING	BATHING	EATING	GETTING DRESSED
Self				
With Help				
Caregiver				

MEALS

BREAKFAST	LUNCH	DINNER
TIME		

SNACKS

AM SNACKS	PM SNACKS

OTHERS

DRINKS	OTHERS

DAILY CARE

TIME	MEDICATION TAKEN

BUSY TIME

PHONE CALLS & VISITS	ACTIVITIES

DOCTORS VISIT

SPECIALIST	COMMENTS

PHYSICAL PAIN

PAIN LOCATION	MARK 1-5

VITALS

	MORNING	MID-DAY	NIGHT
Blood Sugar			
Blood Pressure			
Oxygen Level			
Heart Rate			

OVERALL

HOW WAS THE DAY?

AWESOME	GOOD	OK	DOWN	PAINFUL

REMARKS

WATER INTAKE

SLEEP

TOILET

URINE					
BOWEL					

NOTES

NOTES

☑ **DATE**

DAILY CARE	✓	GROOMING	BATHING	EATING	GETTING DRESSED
	Self				
	With Help				
	Caregiver				

MEALS	BREAKFAST		LUNCH	DINNER
	TIME			

SNACKS	AM SNACKS	PM SNACKS

OTHERS	DRINKS	OTHERS

DAILY CARE	TIME	MEDICATION TAKEN

BUSY TIME	PHONE CALLS & VISITS	ACTIVITIES

	WATER INTAKE	
	SLEEP	

TOILET	URINE					
	BOWEL					
	NOTES					

DOCTORS VISIT	SPECIALIST	COMMENTS

NOTES

PHYSICAL PAIN	PAIN LOCATION	MARK 1-5

VITALS		MORNING	MID-DAY	NIGHT
	Blood Sugar			
	Blood Pressure			
	Oxygen Level			
	Heart Rate			

OVERALL

HOW WAS THE DAY?

AWESOME	GOOD	OK	DOWN	PAINFUL

REMARKS	

DATE [ ]

DAILY CARE	✓	GROOMING	BATHING	EATING	GETTING DRESSED
	Self				
	With Help				
	Caregiver				

MEALS	BREAKFAST	LUNCH	DINNER
TIME			

SNACKS	AM SNACKS	PM SNACKS

OTHERS	DRINKS	OTHERS

DAILY CARE	TIME	MEDICATION TAKEN

BUSY TIME	PHONE CALLS & VISITS	ACTIVITIES

DOCTORS VISIT	SPECIALIST	COMMENTS

PHYSICAL PAIN	PAIN LOCATION	MARK 1-5

VITALS	MORNING	MID-DAY	NIGHT
Blood Sugar			
Blood Pressure			
Oxygen Level			
Heart Rate			

OVERALL

HOW WAS THE DAY?

☺ AWESOME   🙂 GOOD   😐 OK   🙁 DOWN   😣 PAINFUL

REMARKS	

WATER INTAKE

SLEEP

TOILET	URINE					
	BOWEL					

NOTES

NOTES

☑ DATE [   ]

DAILY CARE	✓	GROOMING	BATHING	EATING	GETTING DRESSED
	Self				
	With Help				
	Caregiver				

MEALS	BREAKFAST		LUNCH	DINNER
	TIME			

SNACKS	AM SNACKS	PM SNACKS

OTHERS	DRINKS	OTHERS

DAILY CARE	TIME	MEDICATION TAKEN

BUSY TIME	PHONE CALLS & VISITS	ACTIVITIES

WATER INTAKE

SLEEP

TOILET						
URINE						
BOWEL						
NOTES						

DOCTORS VISIT	SPECIALIST	COMMENTS

NOTES

PHYSICAL PAIN	PAIN LOCATION	MARK 1-5

VITALS	MORNING	MID-DAY	NIGHT
Blood Sugar			
Blood Pressure			
Oxygen Level			
Heart Rate			

OVERALL	HOW WAS THE DAY?
	AWESOME · GOOD · OK · DOWN · PAINFUL
	REMARKS

DATE [ ]

DAILY CARE	✓	GROOMING	BATHING	EATING	GETTING DRESSED
	Self				
	With Help				
	Caregiver				

MEALS	BREAKFAST	LUNCH	DINNER
	TIME		

SNACKS	AM SNACKS	PM SNACKS

OTHERS	DRINKS	OTHERS

DAILY CARE	TIME	MEDICATION TAKEN

BUSY TIME	PHONE CALLS & VISITS	ACTIVITIES

WATER INTAKE

SLEEP

TOILET							
URINE							
BOWEL							
NOTES							

DOCTORS VISIT	SPECIALIST	COMMENTS

NOTES

PHYSICAL PAIN	PAIN LOCATION	MARK 1-5

VITALS		MORNING	MID-DAY	NIGHT
	Blood Sugar			
	Blood Pressure			
	Oxygen Level			
	Heart Rate			

OVERALL	HOW WAS THE DAY?
	☺ AWESOME ☺ GOOD 😐 OK ☹ DOWN ☹ PAINFUL
	REMARKS

DATE

✓	GROOMING	BATHING	EATING	GETTING DRESSED
Self				
With Help				
Caregiver				

DAILY CARE

TIME	BREAKFAST	LUNCH	DINNER

MEALS

AM SNACKS	PM SNACKS

SNACKS

DRINKS	OTHERS

OTHERS

TIME	MEDICATION TAKEN

DAILY CARE

BUSY TIME	PHONE CALLS & VISITS	ACTIVITIES

WATER INTAKE	

SLEEP	

DOCTORS VISIT	SPECIALIST	COMMENTS

TOILET							
URINE							
BOWEL							
NOTES							

PHYSICAL PAIN	PAIN LOCATION	MARK 1-5

NOTES

VITALS		MORNING	MID-DAY	NIGHT
	Blood Sugar			
	Blood Pressure			
	Oxygen Level			
	Heart Rate			

OVERALL	HOW WAS THE DAY?
	AWESOME GOOD OK DOWN PAINFUL
	REMARKS

✓	GROOMING	BATHING	EATING	GETTING DRESSED
Self				
With Help				
Caregiver				

DAILY CARE

BREAKFAST	LUNCH	DINNER
TIME		

MEALS

AM SNACKS	PM SNACKS

SNACKS

DRINKS	OTHERS

OTHERS

TIME	MEDICATION TAKEN

DAILY CARE

BUSY TIME

PHONE CALLS & VISITS	ACTIVITIES

DOCTORS VISIT

SPECIALIST	COMMENTS

PHYSICAL PAIN

PAIN LOCATION	MARK 1-5

VITALS

	MORNING	MID-DAY	NIGHT
Blood Sugar			
Blood Pressure			
Oxygen Level			
Heart Rate			

OVERALL

HOW WAS THE DAY?

AWESOME	GOOD	OK	DOWN	PAINFUL

REMARKS

WATER INTAKE

SLEEP

TOILET

URINE					
BOWEL					

NOTES

NOTES

DATE [ ]

DAILY CARE	✓	GROOMING	BATHING	EATING	GETTING DRESSED
	Self				
	With Help				
	Caregiver				

MEALS		BREAKFAST	LUNCH	DINNER
	TIME			

SNACKS	AM SNACKS	PM SNACKS

OTHERS	DRINKS	OTHERS

DAILY CARE	TIME	MEDICATION TAKEN

BUSY TIME

PHONE CALLS & VISITS	ACTIVITIES

DOCTORS VISIT

SPECIALIST	COMMENTS

PHYSICAL PAIN

PAIN LOCATION	MARK 1-5

VITALS

	MORNING	MID-DAY	NIGHT
Blood Sugar			
Blood Pressure			
Oxygen Level			
Heart Rate			

OVERALL

HOW WAS THE DAY?

:D AWESOME	:) GOOD	:| OK	:(DOWN	>< PAINFUL

REMARKS	

WATER INTAKE

| |

SLEEP

| |

TOILET

URINE						
BOWEL						
NOTES						

NOTES

☑ **DATE** [ ]

DAILY CARE	✓	GROOMING	BATHING	EATING	GETTING DRESSED
	Self				
	With Help				
	Caregiver				

MEALS	BREAKFAST	LUNCH	DINNER
	TIME		

SNACKS	AM SNACKS	PM SNACKS

OTHERS	DRINKS	OTHERS

DAILY CARE	TIME	MEDICATION TAKEN

BUSY TIME	PHONE CALLS & VISITS	ACTIVITIES

	WATER INTAKE	

	SLEEP	

DOCTORS VISIT	SPECIALIST	COMMENTS

TOILET	URINE					
	BOWEL					
	NOTES					

PHYSICAL PAIN	PAIN LOCATION	MARK 1-5

NOTES

VITALS		MORNING	MID-DAY	NIGHT
	Blood Sugar			
	Blood Pressure			
	Oxygen Level			
	Heart Rate			

OVERALL	HOW WAS THE DAY?

AWESOME · GOOD · OK · DOWN · PAINFUL

REMARKS

☑ DATE [ ]

DAILY CARE

✓	GROOMING	BATHING	EATING	GETTING DRESSED
Self				
With Help				
Caregiver				

MEALS

BREAKFAST	LUNCH	DINNER
TIME		

SNACKS

AM SNACKS	PM SNACKS

OTHERS

DRINKS	OTHERS

DAILY CARE

TIME	MEDICATION TAKEN

BUSY TIME	PHONE CALLS & VISITS	ACTIVITIES

WATER INTAKE

SLEEP

TOILET							
URINE							
BOWEL							
NOTES							

DOCTORS VISIT	SPECIALIST	COMMENTS

NOTES

PHYSICAL PAIN	PAIN LOCATION	MARK 1-5

VITALS		MORNING	MID-DAY	NIGHT
	Blood Sugar			
	Blood Pressure			
	Oxygen Level			
	Heart Rate			

OVERALL	HOW WAS THE DAY?
	AWESOME GOOD OK DOWN PAINFUL
	REMARKS

DATE [ ]

DAILY CARE	✓	GROOMING	BATHING	EATING	GETTING DRESSED
	Self				
	With Help				
	Caregiver				

MEALS	BREAKFAST	LUNCH	DINNER
	TIME		

SNACKS	AM SNACKS	PM SNACKS

OTHERS	DRINKS	OTHERS

DAILY CARE	TIME	MEDICATION TAKEN

BUSY TIME	PHONE CALLS & VISITS	ACTIVITIES

WATER INTAKE [ ]

SLEEP [ ]

TOILET							
URINE							
BOWEL							
NOTES							

DOCTORS VISIT	SPECIALIST	COMMENTS

NOTES

PHYSICAL PAIN	PAIN LOCATION	MARK 1-5

VITALS		MORNING	MID-DAY	NIGHT
	Blood Sugar			
	Blood Pressure			
	Oxygen Level			
	Heart Rate			

OVERALL	HOW WAS THE DAY?
	AWESOME GOOD OK DOWN PAINFUL
	REMARKS

☑ DATE [　　　　　　]

DAILY CARE ✓		GROOMING	BATHING	EATING	GETTING DRESSED
	Self				
	With Help				
	Caregiver				

MEALS	BREAKFAST	LUNCH	DINNER
TIME			

SNACKS	AM SNACKS	PM SNACKS

OTHERS	DRINKS	OTHERS

DAILY CARE	TIME	MEDICATION TAKEN

BUSY TIME	PHONE CALLS & VISITS	ACTIVITIES

WATER INTAKE	

SLEEP	

TOILET						
URINE						
BOWEL						
NOTES						

DOCTORS VISIT	SPECIALIST	COMMENTS

PHYSICAL PAIN	PAIN LOCATION	MARK 1-5

NOTES

VITALS		MORNING	MID-DAY	NIGHT
	Blood Sugar			
	Blood Pressure			
	Oxygen Level			
	Heart Rate			

OVERALL	HOW WAS THE DAY?
	AWESOME GOOD OK DOWN PAINFUL
	REMARKS

☑ **DATE** [_____]

DAILY CARE	✓	GROOMING	BATHING	EATING	GETTING DRESSED
	Self				
	With Help				
	Caregiver				

MEALS	BREAKFAST	LUNCH	DINNER
	TIME		

SNACKS	AM SNACKS	PM SNACKS

OTHERS	DRINKS	OTHERS

DAILY CARE	TIME	MEDICATION TAKEN

BUSY TIME

PHONE CALLS & VISITS	ACTIVITIES

DOCTORS VISIT

SPECIALIST	COMMENTS

PHYSICAL PAIN

PAIN LOCATION	MARK 1-5

VITALS

	MORNING	MID-DAY	NIGHT
Blood Sugar			
Blood Pressure			
Oxygen Level			
Heart Rate			

OVERALL

HOW WAS THE DAY?

😃	🙂	😐	🙁	😣
AWESOME	GOOD	OK	DOWN	PAINFUL

REMARKS	

WATER INTAKE

SLEEP

TOILET

URINE					
BOWEL					

NOTES

NOTES

☑ DATE [ ]

DAILY CARE

✓	GROOMING	BATHING	EATING	GETTING DRESSED
Self				
With Help				
Caregiver				

MEALS

BREAKFAST	LUNCH	DINNER
TIME		

SNACKS

AM SNACKS	PM SNACKS

OTHERS

DRINKS	OTHERS

DAILY CARE

TIME	MEDICATION TAKEN

BUSY TIME

PHONE CALLS & VISITS	ACTIVITIES

DOCTORS VISIT

SPECIALIST	COMMENTS

PHYSICAL PAIN

PAIN LOCATION	MARK 1-5

VITALS

	MORNING	MID-DAY	NIGHT
Blood Sugar			
Blood Pressure			
Oxygen Level			
Heart Rate			

OVERALL

HOW WAS THE DAY?

AWESOME	GOOD	OK	DOWN	PAINFUL

REMARKS	

WATER INTAKE

SLEEP

TOILET

URINE					
BOWEL					

NOTES

NOTES

☑ **DATE**

DAILY CARE	✓	GROOMING	BATHING	EATING	GETTING DRESSED
	Self				
	With Help				
	Caregiver				

MEALS	BREAKFAST	LUNCH	DINNER
	TIME		

SNACKS	AM SNACKS	PM SNACKS

OTHERS	DRINKS	OTHERS

DAILY CARE	TIME	MEDICATION TAKEN

BUSY TIME	PHONE CALLS & VISITS	ACTIVITIES

	WATER INTAKE	
	SLEEP	

DOCTORS VISIT	SPECIALIST	COMMENTS

TOILET	URINE					
	BOWEL					
	NOTES					

PHYSICAL PAIN	PAIN LOCATION	MARK 1-5

NOTES

VITALS		MORNING	MID-DAY	NIGHT
	Blood Sugar			
	Blood Pressure			
	Oxygen Level			
	Heart Rate			

OVERALL	HOW WAS THE DAY?
	AWESOME GOOD OK DOWN PAINFUL
	REMARKS

ADDITIONAL NOTES

Made in the USA
Monee, IL
26 December 2022

23694454R00063